Healthy Keto Vegetarian Recipes

Lose Weight and Feel Great with these Easy to Cook Plant-Based Keto Vegetarian Recipes

Dr. William Coleman

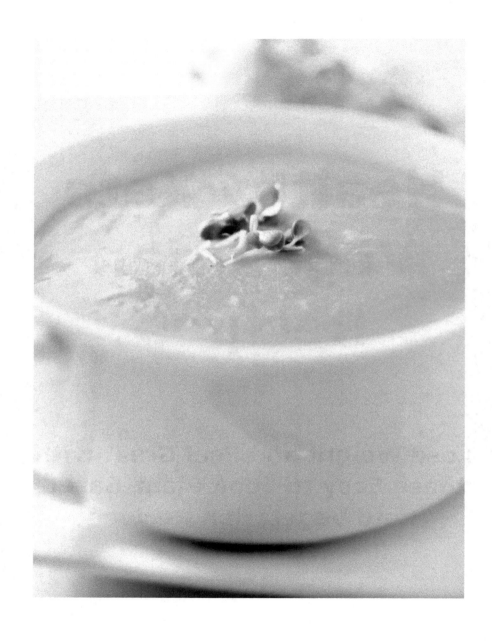

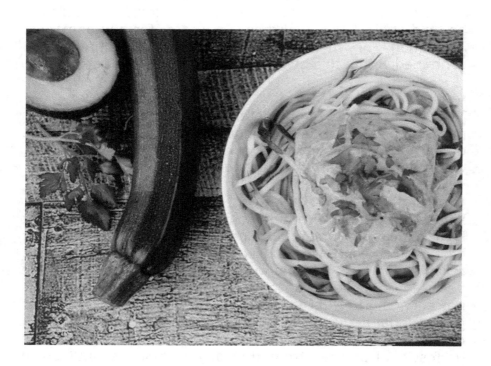

TABLE OF CONTENTS

INTRODUCTION 1

Mint Watermelon Bowl 3

Classic French Toasts 5

Raspberry, Hazelnut and Pecan Porridge 8

Bok Choy Salad 10

Creamy Coconut Curry 12

Avocado Cilantro Tomato Salad 14

Keto Tofu and Spinach Casserole 15

Healthy Braised Garlic Kale 17

Spinach Tomato Stir Fry 19

Spinach Mix 21

Quinoa with Olives 23

Thai Veggie Mix 25

Lemon Garlic Mushrooms 27

Mozzarella Cheese (vegan) 29

Sage Pecan Cauliflower 31

Roasted Cauliflower Tacos 33

Cajun Sweet Potatoes 36

Broccoli With Almonds 38

Miso Spaghetti Squash 40

Grilled Artichokes 42

Artichokes and Tomatoes Dip 44

Fresh Fruit Smoothie........................... 46

Radish Soup.................................... 47

Easy Corn Chowder.............................. 49

Squash Soup With Pecans And Ginger 51

Hot & Sour Tofu Soup 53

Root Vegetable Soup............................ 55

Avocado Broccoli Soup 57

Zoodle Bolognese 59

Delicious Sambal Seitan Noodles 62

Romaine And Grape Tomato Salad With Avocado
And Baby Peas 65

Quick And Easy Ranch Dip 67

Queso Blanco Dip 69

Tempeh-Pimiento Cheeze Ball 71

Coconut Rice................................... 73

Rice Pizza 75

Quinoa and Black Bean Burgers.................. 77

Cinnamon Bun Balls............................. 79

Strawberry Shortcake Chaffle Bowls................. 80

Mint Chocolate Chip Sorbet...............................82

Tangerine Stew...84

Pineapple and Melon Stew 85

Avocado and Rhubarb Salad 86

Vanilla Raspberries Mix 87

Sweet Zucchini Buns...88

Lime Berries Stew 90

Apricots Cake 91

Nutmeg Pudding 93

Avocado and Almond Sweet Cream 95

Chia Bowls 96

Cocoa Cream 97

Raspberry Protein Shake (vegan) 99

NOTE **101**

INTRODUCTION

Essentially, a ketogenic diet is a diet that drastically restricts your carb intake and fat intake; this pushes your body to go into a state of ketosis.

Your body uses glucose from carbs to fuel metabolic pathways—meaning various bodily functions like digestion, breathing—essentially anything that needs energy. Glucose is therefore the primary pathway when it comes to sourcing the body's energy.

But the body has also another pathway, it can make use of fats to fuel the various bodily processes. And this is what is called ketosis. The body can only enter ketosis when there is no glucose available, thus the reason why eating a low-carb diet is essential in the keto diet.

Since no glucose is available, the body is pushed to use fats—it can either come from the food you consume or from your body's fat reserves—the adipose tissue or from the flabby parts of your body. This is how the keto diet helps you lose weight, by burning up all those stored fats that you have and using it to fuel bodily processes.

Ketosis is a very natural process, the body will soon adapt to this state and therefore you will be able to lose weight in no time but you will also become healthier and your physical and mental performances will improve. Your blood sugar levels will improve and you won't be predisposed to diabetes. Also, epilepsy and heart disease can be easily be prevented if you are on a ketogenic diet. Your cholesterol will improve and you will feel amazing in no time. How does that sound?

That said, if for whatever reason you are a vegetarian, following a ketogenic diet can be extremely difficult. A vegetarian diet is largely free of animal products, which means that food tends to be usually high in carbohydrates. Still, with careful planning, it is possible.

This Cookbook will provide you with various easy and delicious dishes to help you stick to your ketogenic diet plan while being a vegetarian.

Enjoy!

Mint Watermelon Bowl

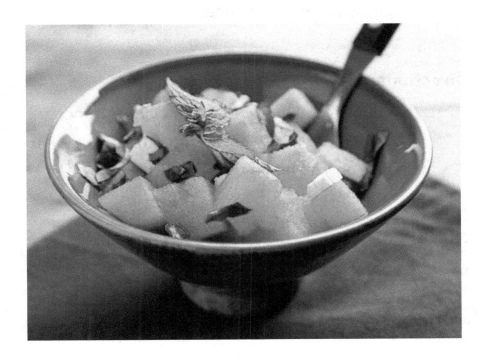

Preparation time: 5 minutes

Cooking time: 0 minutes

Servings: 2

Ingredients:

- 2 cups watermelon, peeled and cubed
- 6 kalamata olives, pitted and sliced

- 1 teaspoon avocado oil
- ½ tablespoon balsamic vinegar
- 1 tablespoon mint, chopped

Directions:

1. In a bowl, combine the watermelon with the olives and the other ingredients, toss, divide into smaller bowls and serve.

Nutrition:

calories 90, fat 3, fiber 1, carbs 7, protein 2

Classic French Toasts

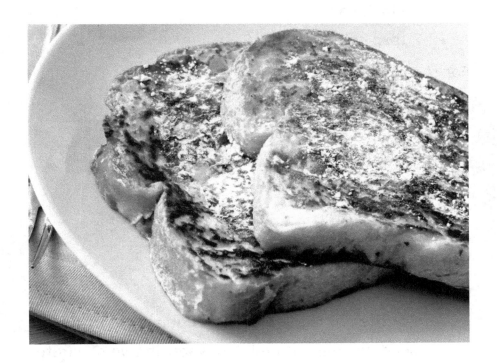

Preparation Time: 10 minutes

Cooking Time: 6 minutes

Serving: 6 minutes

Ingredients:

For the glass dish bread:

- 2 tbsp flax seed meal + 6 tbsp water
- 1 tsp butter
- 2 tbsp coconut flour

- 2 tbsp almond flour
- 1½ tsp baking powder
- A pinch salt
- 2 tbsp coconut cream

For the toast's batter:

- 2 tbsp flax seed meal + 6 tbsp water
- 2 tbsp coconut milk
- ½ tsp cinnamon powder + extra for garnishing
- 1 pinch salt
- 2 tbsp butter

Directions:

For the glass dish bread:

1. For the flax egg, whisk both quantities of flax seed powder with mixing water in two separate bowls and leave to soak for 5 minutes.
2. Then, grease a glass dish (for the microwave) with the butter.
3. In another bowl, mix the coconut flour, almond flour, baking powder, and salt.
4. When the flax seed egg is ready, whisk one portion with the coconut cream and add the mixture to the dry Ingredients.
5. Continue whisking until the mixture is smooth with no lumps.

6. Pour the dough into the glass dish and microwave for 2 minutes or until the middle part of the bread is done.
7. Take out and allow the bread to cool. Then, remove the bread and slice in half. Return to the glass dish.

For the toast:

8. Whisk the mixture the remaining flax egg with the coconut cream, cinnamon powder, and salt until well combined.
9. Pour the mixture over the bread slices and leave to soak. Turn the bread a few times to soak in as much of the batter.
10. Next, melt the butter in a frying pan and fry the bread slices in the butter on both sides.
11. When golden brown on both sides, transfer the bread to a serving plate, sprinkle with cinnamon powder, and serve immediately with a cup of tea or bulletproof coffee.

Nutrition:

Calories: 96, Total Fat: 9.9g, Saturated Fat: 6.7g, Total Carbs: 2g, Dietary Fiber: 1g, Sugar: 1g, Protein: 1g, Sodium: 66mg

Raspberry, Hazelnut and Pecan Porridge

Preparation Time: 8 minutes

Cooking Time: 15 minutes

Serving: 2

Ingredients:

- 2 tbsp coconut flour
- 1 tsp psyllium husk powder
- Salt to taste
- 6 tbsp coconut cream
- 2 oz butter
- 2 eggs
- 2 tbsp freshly squeezed lemon juice
- 1 tsp cinnamon powder
- 6 fresh raspberries, halved
- 4 tbsp chopped hazelnuts
- 2 tbsp chopped pecans

Directions:

1. In a medium saucepan, combine the coconut flour, psyllium husk powder, salt, coconut cream, egg, lemon juice, and cinnamon powder.

2. Cook the Ingredients over low heat while stirring constantly but do not allow boiling until thickened.
3. Dish the porridge and top with the raspberries, hazelnuts, and pecans. Serve warm.

Nutrition:

Calories: 96, Total Fat: 9.9g, Saturated Fat:6.7 g, Total Carbs: 2 g, Dietary Fiber: 1, Sugar: 1g, Protein: 1g, Sodium: 66mg

Bok Choy Salad

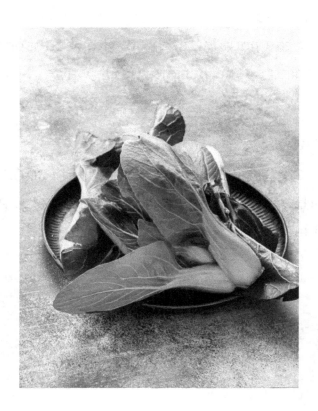

Preparation time: 10 minutes

Cooking time: 20 minutes

Servings: 4

Ingredients:

- 4 scallions, chopped

- 1 pound bok choy, torn
- 2 tablespoons olive oil
- ½ cup veggie stock
- 2 tablespoons balsamic vinegar
- 1 tablespoon chili powder
- 1 cup cherry tomatoes, halved
- 1 tablespoon garlic powder
- ¼ cup chives, chopped
- 1 teaspoon rosemary, dried
- 1 tablespoon thyme, chopped
- A pinch of sea salt and black pepper

Directions:

1. Heat up a pan with the oil over medium heat, add the scallions, garlic powder and rosemary, stir and cook for 5 minutes.
2. Add the bok choy and the rest of the ingredients, toss, cook over medium heat for 15 minutes, divide between plates and serve.

Nutrition:

calories 107, fat 8.4, fiber 3.4, carbs 9, protein 3.1

Creamy Coconut Curry

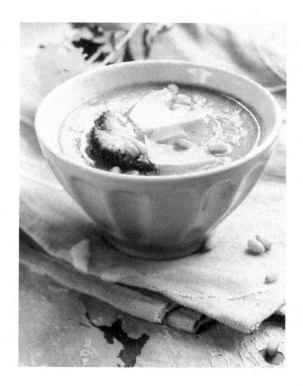

Preparation Time: 15 minutes

Cooking Time: 30 minutes

Servings: 4

Ingredients:

- 1 teaspoon garlic, minced
- 1 teaspoon ginger, minced

- 2 teaspoons soy sauce
- 1 tablespoon red curry paste
- 1 cup broccoli florets
- 1 handful spinach
- ¼ of an onion, sliced
- ½ cup coconut cream
- 4 tablespoons coconut oil

Directions:

1. In a saucepan over medium-high heat, heat your coconut oil. Add your onion to the pan and cook until softened. Add garlic and cook until lightly browned. Reduce heat to medium-low, adding broccoli, stir well. Cook for about 20 minutes then add the curry paste and stir. Add spinach over broccoli and cook until wilted. Add soy sauce, ginger and coconut cream, and stir. Simmer for an additional 10 minutes. Serve hot and enjoy!

Nutritional Values (Per Serving):

Calories: 235 Cholesterol: 0 mg Sugar: 2.1 g
Carbohydrates: 8.4 g Fat: 22.3 g Protein: 4.1 g

Avocado Cilantro Tomato Salad

Preparation Time: 15 minutes

Servings: 4

Ingredients:

- 4 cups cherry tomatoes, halved
- 2 avocados, diced
- Juice of 1 lime, fresh
- ¼ cup cilantro, fresh, chopped
- 1 tablespoon extra-virgin olive oil
- Pepper and salt to taste

Directions:

1. In a mixing bowl add tomatoes, avocado, and cilantro. In a small bowl, combine lime juice, olive oil, pepper, and salt. Pour lime juice mixture over salad and mix well. Enjoy!

Nutritional Values (Per Serving):

Calories: 270 Fat: 23.5 g Cholesterol: 0 mg Sugar: 5.4 g Carbohydrates: 16.6 g Protein: 3.6 g

Keto Tofu and Spinach Casserole

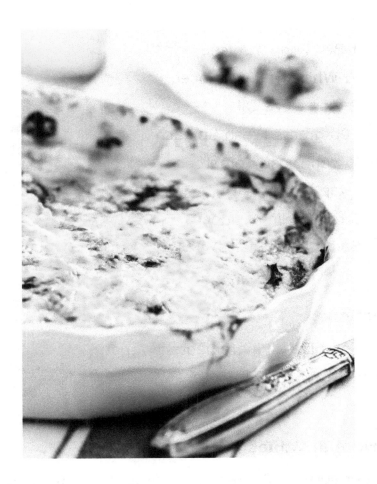

Preparation Time: 5 min

Cooking Time: 5 min

Serves: 4

Ingredients:

- 1 block Firm Tofu, drained, pressed, and cut into cubes
- 1 Bell Pepper, diced
- ½ White Onion, minced
- 2 tbsp Olive Oil
- 100 grams Fresh Spinach
- ½ cup Diced Tomatoes
- 1 tsp Paprika
- 1 tsp Garlic Powder
- Salt and Pepper to taste

Directions:

1. Combine all ingredients in a pot.
2. Simmer for 5 minutes

Nutritional Values:

Kcal per serve: 222 Fat: 15 g. Protein: 17 g. Carbs: 7 g.

Healthy Braised Garlic Kale

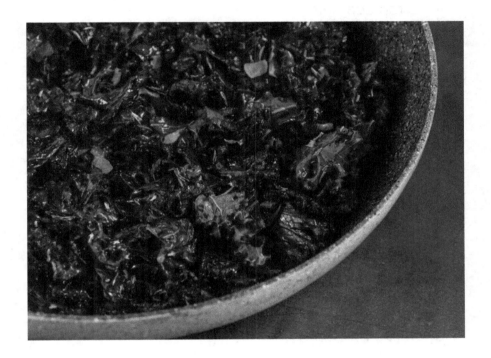

Preparation Time: 50 minutes

Servings: 4

Ingredients:

- 10 oz kale, stems removed and chopped
- 2 cups vegetable stock
- 4 tbsp coconut oil
- 1 tsp chili pepper flakes, dried

- 1 medium onion, sliced
- 4 garlic cloves, minced
- 1 tsp sea salt

Directions:

1. Heat coconut oil in a pan over medium heat.
2. Once the oil is hot then add onion, garlic and chili pepper flakes and sauté until lightly brown.
3. Pour vegetable stock and stir well.
4. Now add chopped kale and season with salt. Stir well.
5. Cover pan with lid and cook on low heat for 40 minutes.
6. Serve and enjoy.

Nutritional Value (Amount per Serving):

Calories 172 Fat 14 g Carbohydrates 11 g Sugar 1 g Protein 2 g Cholesterol 0 mg

Spinach Tomato Stir Fry

Preparation Time: 10 minutes

Cooking Time: 15 minutes

Servings: 2

Ingredients:

- 1/2 cup cherry tomatoes, cut in half
- 1/2 onion, sliced
- 4 cups spinach
- 1 garlic clove, diced
- 1/2 tsp lemon zest
- 2 tsp olive oil
- 6 button mushrooms, sliced
- Pepper
- Salt

Directions:

1. Heat olive oil in a pan over medium heat.
2. Add mushrooms and sauté for 3-4 minutes or until lightly browned.
3. Remove mushrooms to a plate and set aside.
4. Add onion and sauté for 2-3 minutes or until

softened.

5. Add tomatoes, garlic and lemon zest, and season with pepper and salt. Cook for 2-3 minutes and lightly smashed tomatoes with a spatula.

6. Now add mushrooms and spinach and stir well and cook until spinach is wilted.

7. Season with salt and drizzle with lemon juice.

8. Serve and enjoy.

Nutrition:

Calories 104 Fat 7.1 g Carbohydrates 8.9 g Sugar 3.6 g Protein 4.3 g Cholesterol 5 mg

Spinach Mix

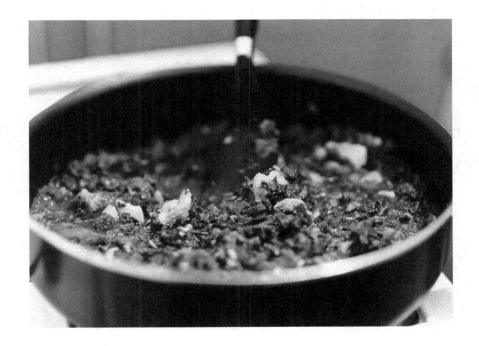

Preparation time: 10 minutes

Cooking time: 12 minutes

Servings: 4

Ingredients:

- 1 pound baby spinach
- 1 yellow onion, chopped
- 1 tablespoon olive oil

- 1 tablespoon lemon juice
- 2 garlic cloves, minced
- A pinch of cayenne pepper
- ¼ teaspoon smoked paprika
- A pinch of salt and black pepper

Directions:

1. Heat up a pan with the oil over medium-high heat, add the onion and the garlic and sauté for 2 minutes.
2. Add the spinach and the other ingredients, toss, cook over medium heat for 10 minutes, divide between plates and serve as a side dish.

Nutrition:

calories 71, fat 4, fiber 3.2, carbs 7.4, protein 3.7

Quinoa with Olives

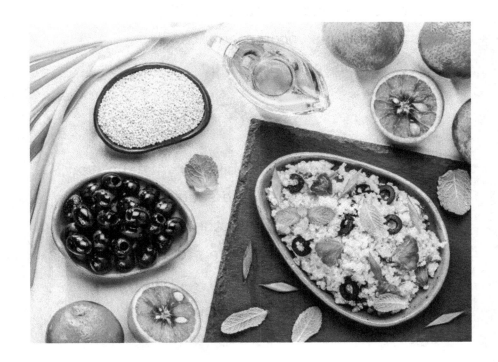

Preparation time: 10 minutes

Cooking time: 30 minutes

Servings: 4

Ingredients:

- 1 yellow onion, chopped
- 1 tablespoon olive oil
- 1 cup quinoa

- 3 cups vegetable stock
- ½ cup black olives, pitted and halved
- 2 green onions, chopped
- 2 tablespoons coconut aminos
- 1 teaspoon rosemary, dried

Directions:

1. Heat up a pot with the oil over medium heat, add the yellow onion and sauté for 5 minutes.
2. Add the quinoa and the other ingredients except the green onions, stir, bring to a simmer and cook over medium heat for 25 minutes.
3. Divide the mix between plates, sprinkle the green onions on top and serve.

Nutrition:

calories 261, fat 6, fiber 8, carbs 10, protein 6

Thai Veggie Mix

Preparation time: 10 minutes

Cooking time: 3 hours

Servings: 8

Ingredients:

- 8 ounces yellow summer squash, peeled and roughly chopped
- 12 ounces zucchini, halved and sliced
- 2 cups button mushrooms, quartered
- 1 red sweet potatoes, chopped
- 2 leeks, sliced
- 2 tablespoons veggie stock
- 2 garlic cloves, minced
- 2 tablespoon Thai red curry paste
- 1 tablespoon ginger, grated
- 1/3 cup coconut milk
- ¼ cup basil, chopped

Directions:

1. In your slow cooker, mix zucchini with summer squash, mushrooms, red pepper, leeks, garlic,

stock, curry paste, ginger, coconut milk and basil, toss, cover and cook on Low for 3 hours.

2. Stir your Thai mix one more time, divide between plates and serve as a side dish.

3. Enjoy!

Nutrition:

calories 69, fat 2, fiber 2, carbs 8, protein 2

Lemon Garlic Mushrooms

Preparation Time: 10 minutes

Cooking Time: 15 minutes

Servings: 4

Ingredients:

- 3 oz enoki mushrooms
- 1 tbsp olive oil
- 1 tsp lemon zest, chopped
- 2 tbsp lemon juice
- 3 garlic cloves, sliced
- 6 oyster mushrooms, halved
- 5 oz cremini mushrooms, sliced
- 1/2 red chili, sliced
- 1/2 onion, sliced
- 1 tsp sea salt

Directions:

1. Heat olive oil in a pan over high heat.
2. Add shallots, enoki mushrooms, oyster mushrooms, cremini mushrooms, and chili.
3. Stir well and cook over medium-high heat for 10

minutes.

4. Add lemon zest and stir well. Season with lemon juice and salt and cook for 3-4 minutes.
5. Serve and enjoy.

Nutrition:

Calories 87 Fat 5.6 g Carbohydrates 7.5 g Sugar 1.8 g Protein 3 g Cholesterol 8 mg

Mozzarella Cheese (vegan)

Preparation time: 20 minutes

Cooking time: 0 minute

Servings: 16

Ingredients:

- 1 cup raw cashews (unsalted)
- ½ cup macadamia nuts (unsalted)
- ½ cup pine nuts
- ½ cup water
- ½ tbsp. coconut oil
- ½ tsp. light miso paste
- 2 tbsp. agar-agar
- 1 tsp. fresh lime juice
- 1 tsp. Himalayan salt

Directions:

1. Cover the cashews with water in a small bowl and let sit for 4 to 6 hours. Rinse and drain the cashews after soaking. Make sure no water is left.
2. Mix the agar-agar with the ½ cup of water in a small saucepan. Put the pan over medium heat.
3. Bring the agar-agar mixture to a boil. After 1

minute, take it off the heat and set the mixture aside to cool down.

4. Put all the other ingredients—except the coconut oil—in a blender or food processor. Blend until everything is well combined.

5. Add the agar-agar with water and blend again until all ingredients have been fully incorporated.

6. Grease a medium-sized bowl with the coconut oil to prevent the cheese from sticking to the edges. Gently transfer the cheese mixture into the bowl by using a spatula.

7. Refrigerate the bowl, uncovered, for about 3 hours until the cheese is firm; then serve and enjoy!

8. Alternatively, store the cheese in an airtight container in the fridge. Consume within 6 days. Store for a maximum of 60 days in the freezer and thaw at room temperature.

Nutrition:

Calories: 101kcal, Net Carbs: 2.1g, Fat: 9.2g, Protein: 2.2g, Fiber: 0.9g, Sugar: 0.9g

Sage Pecan Cauliflower

Preparation Time: 10 minutes

Cooking Time: 30 minutes

Servings: 6

Ingredients:

- 1 large cauliflower head, cut into florets
- 1/2 tsp dried thyme
- 1/2 tsp poultry seasoning
- 1/4 cup olive oil
- 2 garlic clove, minced
- 1/4 cup pecans, chopped
- 2 tbsp parsley, chopped
- 1/2 tsp ground sage
- 1/4 cup celery, chopped
- 1 onion, sliced
- 1/4 tsp black pepper
- 1 tsp sea salt

Directions:

1. Preheat the oven to 450 F/ 232 C.

2. Spray a baking tray with cooking spray and set aside.
3. In a large bowl, mix together cauliflower, thyme, poultry seasoning, olive oil, garlic, celery, sage, onions, pepper, and salt.
4. Spread mixture on a baking tray and roast in preheated oven for 15 minutes.
5. Add pecans and parsley and stir well. Roast for 10-15 minutes more.
6. Serve and enjoy.

Nutrition:

Calories 118, Fat 8.6g, Carbohydrates 9.9g, Sugar 4.2g, Protein 3.1g, Cholesterol 0mg

Roasted Cauliflower Tacos

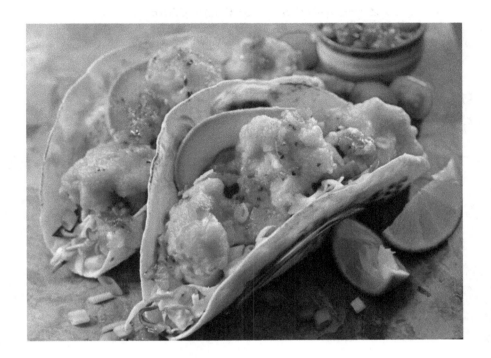

Preparation time: 10 minutes

cooking time: 30 minutes

Servings: 8 TACOS

Ingredients

For the roasted cauliflower

- 1 head cauliflower, cut into bite-size pieces
- 1 tablespoon olive oil (optional

- 2 tablespoons whole-wheat flour
- 2 tablespoons nutritional yeast
- 1 to 2 teaspoons smoked paprika
- ½ to 1 teaspoon chili powder
- Pinch sea salt

For the tacos

- 2 cups shredded lettuce
- 2 cups cherry tomatoes, quartered
- 2 carrots, scrubbed or peeled, and grated
- ½ cup Fresh Mango Salsa
- ½ cup Guacamole
- 8 small whole-grain or corn tortillas
- 1 lime, cut into 8 wedges

Directions

To Make The Roasted Cauliflower

1. Preheat the oven to 350°F. Lightly grease a large rectangular baking sheet with olive oil, or line it with parchment paper.
2. In a large bowl, toss the cauliflower pieces with oil (if using), or just rinse them so they're wet.

3. The idea is to get the seasonings to stick. In a smaller bowl, mix together the flour, nutritional yeast, paprika, chili powder, and salt.
4. Add the seasonings to the cauliflower, and mix it around with your hands to thoroughly coat. Spread the cauliflower on the baking sheet, and roast for 20 to 30 minutes, or until softened.

To Make The Tacos.

5. Prep the veggies, salsa, and guacamole while the cauliflower is roasting.
6. Once the cauliflower is cooked, heat the tortillas for just a few minutes in the oven or in a small skillet.
7. Set everything out on the table, and assemble your tacos as you go.
8. Give a squeeze of fresh lime just before eating.

Nutrition (1 taco):

Calories: 198; Total fat: 6g; Carbs: 32g; Fiber: 6g; Protein: 7g

Cajun Sweet Potatoes

Preparation time: 5 minutes

cooking time: 30 minutes

servings: 4

Ingredients

- 2 pounds sweet potatoes
- 2 teaspoons extra-virgin olive oil
- ½ teaspoon ground cayenne pepper
- ½ teaspoon smoked paprika
- ½ teaspoon dried oregano
- ½ teaspoon dried thyme
- ½ teaspoon garlic powder
- ½ teaspoon salt (optional)

Directions

1. Preheat the oven to 400ºF. Line a baking sheet with parchment paper.
2. Wash the potatoes, pat dry, and cut into ¾-inch cubes. Transfer to a large bowl, and pour the olive oil over the potatoes.

3. In a small bowl, combine the cayenne, paprika, oregano, thyme, and garlic powder.
4. Sprinkle the spices over the potatoes and combine until the potatoes are well coated. Spread the potatoes on the prepared baking sheet in a single layer.
5. Season with the salt (if using). Roast for 30 minutes, stirring the potatoes after 15 minutes.
6. Divide the potatoes evenly among 4 single-serving containers. Let cool completely before sealing.

Nutrition:

Calories: 219; Fat: 3g; Protein: 4g; Carbohydrates: 46g; Fiber: 7g; Sugar: 9g; Sodium: 125mg

Broccoli With Almonds

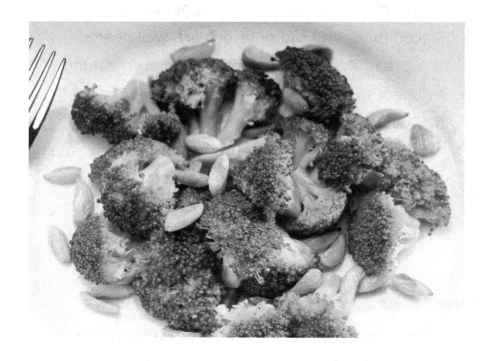

Preparation time: 5 minutes

cooking time: 15 minutes

servings: 4

Ingredients

- 1 pound broccoli, cut into small florets
- 2 tablespoons olive oil
- 3 garlic cloves, minced

- 1 cup thinly sliced white mushrooms
- 1/4 cup dry white wine
- 2 tablespoons minced fresh parsley
- Salt and freshly ground black pepper
- 1/2 cup slivered toasted almonds

Directions

1. Steam the broccoli until just tender, about 5 minutes. Run under cold water and set aside.
2. In a large skillet, heat 1 tablespoon of the oil over medium heat. Add the garlic and mushrooms and cook until soft, about 5 minutes. Add the wine and cook 1 minute longer. Add the steamed broccoli and parsley and season with salt and pepper to taste. Cook until the liquid is evaporated and the broccoli is hot, about 3 minutes.
3. Transfer to a serving bowl, drizzle with the remaining 1 tablespoon oil and the almonds, and toss to coat. Serve immediately.

Miso Spaghetti Squash

Preparation time: 5 minutes

cooking time: 40 minutes

servings: 4

Ingredients

- 1 (3-poundspaghetti squash
- 1 tablespoon hot water
- 1 tablespoon unseasoned rice vinegar
- 1 tablespoon white miso

Directions

1. Preheat the oven to 400ºF. Line a rimmed baking sheet with parchment paper.
2. Halve the squash lengthwise and place, cut-side down, on the prepared baking sheet.
3. Bake for 35 to 40 minutes, until tender. Cool until the squash is easy to handle. With a fork, scrape out the flesh, which will be stringy, like spaghetti.
4. Transfer to a large bowl.

5. In a small bowl, combine the hot water, vinegar, and miso with a whisk or fork. Pour over the squash.
6. Gently toss with tongs to coat the squash.
7. Divide the squash evenly among 4 single-serving containers.
8. Let cool before sealing the lids.

Nutrition:

Calories: 117; Fat: 2g; Protein: 3g; Carbohydrates: 25g; Fiber: 0g; Sugar: 0g; Sodium: 218mg

Grilled Artichokes

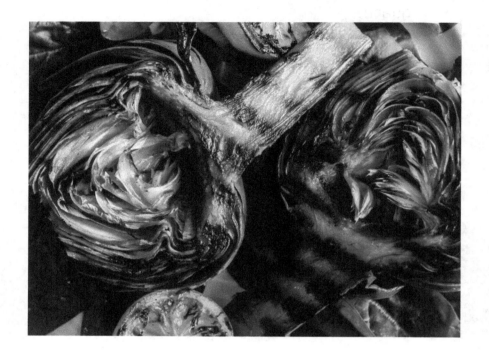

Preparation time: 10 minutes

Cooking time: 25 minutes

Servings: 4

Ingredients:

- 2 artichokes, trimmed and halved
- Juice of 1 lemon
- 1 tablespoons lemon zest grated

- 1 rosemary spring, chopped
- 2 tablespoons olive oil
- A pinch of sea salt
- Black pepper to taste

Directions:

1. Put water in a large saucepan, add a pinch of salt and lemon juice, bring to a boil over medium-high heat, add artichokes, boil for 15 minutes, drain and leave them to cool down.
2. Drizzle olive oil over them, season with black pepper to taste, sprinkle lemon zest and rosemary, stir well and place them under a preheated grill.
3. Broil artichokes over medium-high heat for 5 minutes on each side, divide them between plates and serve.
4. Enjoy!

Nutritional value/serving:

calories 98, fat 7,1, fiber 4,4, carbs 8,5, protein 2,7

Artichokes and Tomatoes Dip

Preparation time: 10 minutes

Cooking time: 30 minutes

Servings: 4

Ingredients:

- 2 artichokes, cut in halves and trimmed
- Juice from 3 lemons
- 4 sun-dried tomatoes, chopped
- A bunch of parsley, chopped
- A bunch of basil, chopped
- 1 garlic clove, minced
- 4 tablespoons olive oil
- Black pepper to taste

Directions:

1. In a bowl, mix artichokes with lemon juice from 1 lemon, some black pepper and toss to coat.
2. Transfer to a large saucepan, add water to cover, bring to a boil over medium-high heat, cook for 30 minutes and drain.

3. In a food processor, mix the rest of the lemon juice with tomatoes, parsley, basil, garlic, black pepper and olive oil and blend well.
4. Divide artichokes between plates and top each with the tomatoes dip.
5. Enjoy!

Nutritional value/serving:

calories 193, fat 14,5, fiber 6,1, carbs 16,9, protein 4,1

Fresh Fruit Smoothie

Preparation Time: 5 mins

Servings: 4

Ingredients:

- 1 tbsp. honey
- ½ c. cantaloupe
- 1 c. water
- 1 c. fresh strawberries
- 1 c. fresh pineapple
- 2 orange juice

Directions:

1. Remove the rind from the melon and pineapple. Cut them into chunks and remove the stems from the strawberries.
2. Put everything in a blender and serve.

Nutrition:

Calories: 72, Fat:1 g, Carbs:17 g, Protein:1 g, Sugars:1 g, Sodium:42 mg

Radish Soup

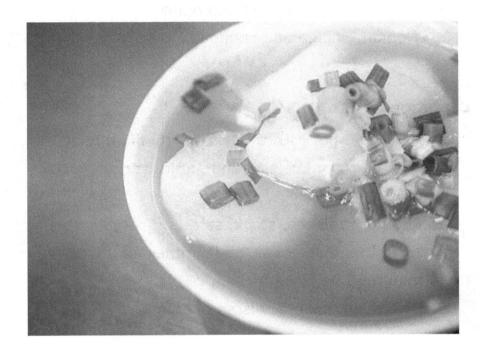

Preparation time: 10 minutes

Cooking time: 20 minutes

Servings: 4

Ingredients:

- 2 bunches radishes, cut in quarters
- Salt and ground black pepper, to taste
- 6 cups chicken stock

- 2 stalks celery, chopped
- 3 tablespoons coconut oil
- 6 garlic cloves, peeled and minced
- 1 onion, peeled and chopped

Directions:

1. Heat up a pot with the oil over medium heat, add the onion, celery, and garlic, stir, and cook for 5 minutes.
2. Add the radishes, stock, salt, and pepper, stir, bring to a boil, cover, and simmer for 15 minutes.
3. Divide into soup bowls and serve.

Nutrition:

Calories - 120, Fat - 2, Fiber - 1, Carbs - 3, Protein - 10

Easy Corn Chowder

Preparation time: 15 minutes

cooking time: 15 minutes

servings: 4

Ingredients

- 2 tablespoons olive oil or other vegetable oil, such as coconut oil
- 1 onion, chopped
- 1 cup chopped fennel bulb or celery
- 2 carrots, peeled and chopped
- 1 red bell pepper, finely chopped
- ¼ cup all-purpose flour
- 6 cups vegetable stock
- 2 cups fresh or canned corn
- 2 cups cubed red potato
- 1 cup unsweetened almond milk or other unsweetened nut or grain milk
- ½ teaspoon sriracha sauce or chili paste (optional
- sea salt
- freshly ground black pepper

Directions

1. In a large pot, heat the olive oil over medium-high heat until it shimmers.
2. Add the onion, fennel, carrots, and bell pepper and cook, stirring occasionally, until the vegetables soften, about 3 minutes.
3. Sprinkle the flour over the vegetables and continue to cook, stirring constantly, for about 2 minutes.
4. Stir in the vegetable stock, using a spoon to scrape any bits of flour or vegetables from the bottom of the pan. Continue stirring until the liquid comes to a boil and the soup begins to thicken. Lower the heat to medium.
5. Add the corn, potatoes, almond milk, and Sriracha, if using. Simmer until the potatoes are soft, about 10 minutes. Season with salt and pepper. Serve hot.

Squash Soup With Pecans And Ginger

Preparation time: 10 minutes

cooking time: 30 minutes

servings: 4

Ingredients

- 1/3 cup toasted pecans
- 2 tablespoons chopped crystallized ginger
- 1 tablespoon canola or grapeseed oil
- 1 medium onion, chopped
- 1 celery rib, chopped
- 1 teaspoon grated fresh ginger
- 5 cups vegetable broth, homemade (see Light Vegetable Brothor store-bought, or water
- 1 kabocha squash, peeled, seeded, and cut into 1/2-inch dice
- 1/4 cup pure maple syrup
- 2 tablespoons soy sauce
- 1/4 teaspoon ground allspice
- Salt and freshly ground black pepper
- 1 cup plain unsweetened soy milk

Directions

1. In a food processor, combine the pecans and crystallized ginger and pulse until coarsely chopped. Set aside.
2. In a large soup pot, heat the oil over medium heat. Add the onion, celery, and fresh ginger. Cover and cook until softened, about 5 minutes. Stir in the broth and squash, cover, and bring to a boil. Reduce the heat to low and simmer, covered, stirring occasionally, until the squash is tender, about 30 minutes.
3. Stir in the maple syrup, soy sauce, allspice, and salt and pepper to taste. Puree in the pot with an immersion blender or in a blender or food processor, in batches if necessary, and return to the pot.
4. Stir in the soy milk and heat over low heat until hot. Ladle the soup into bowls and sprinkle with the pecan and ginger mixture, and serve.

Hot & Sour Tofu Soup

Preparation Time: 40 Minutes

Cooking Time: 15 Minutes

Servings:3

Ingredients

- 6 to 7 ounces firm or extra-firm tofu
- 1 teaspoon olive oil
- 1 cup sliced mushrooms
- 1 cup finely chopped cabbage
- 1 garlic clove, minced
- ½-inch piece fresh ginger, peeled and minced
- Salt
- 4 cups water or Economical Vegetable Broth
- 2 tablespoons rice vinegar or apple cider vinegar
- 2 tablespoons soy sauce
- 1 teaspoon toasted sesame oil
- 1 teaspoon sugar
- Pinch red pepper flakes
- 1 scallion, white and light green parts only, chopped

Directions

1. Preparing the Ingredients.
2. Press your tofu before you start: Put it between several layers of paper towels and place a heavy pan or book (with a waterproof cover or protected with plastic wrap) on top. Let stand for 30 minutes. Discard the paper towels. Cut the tofu into ½-inch cubes.
3. In a large soup pot, heat the olive oil over medium-high heat.
4. Add the mushrooms, cabbage, garlic, ginger, and a pinch of salt. Sauté for 7 to 8 minutes, until the vegetables are softened.
5. Add the water, vinegar, soy sauce, sesame oil, sugar, red pepper flakes, and tofu.
6. Bring to a boil, then turn the heat to low. Simmer the soup for 5 to 10 minutes.
7. Serve with the scallion sprinkled on top.
8. Leftovers will keep in an airtight container for up to 1 week in the refrigerator or up to 1 month in the freezer.

Nutrition Per Serving (2 cups)

Calories: 161; Protein: 13g; Total fat: 9g; Saturated fat: 1g; Carbohydrates: 10g; Fiber: 3g

Root Vegetable Soup

Preparation Time: 15 Minutes

Cooking Time: 15 Minutes

Servings:4

Ingredients

- 2 tablespoons olive oil
- 1 onion, diced
- 3 garlic cloves, minced
- 1 carrot, julienned or grated
- 1 rutabaga, julienned or grated
- 1 parsnip, julienned or grated
- 1 red potato, julienned or grated
- 5 cups vegetable stock
- 2 teaspoons dried thyme
- sea salt
- freshly ground black pepper

Directions

1. In a large soup pot, heat the olive oil over medium-high heat until it shimmers.

2. Add the onion and cook until it softens, about 5 minutes.
3. Add the garlic and cook until it is fragrant, about 30 seconds.
4. Add the carrot, rutabaga, parsnip, potato, vegetable stock, and thyme.
5. Cover and boil until vegetables soften, about 10 minutes.
6. Remove from the heat. Using a food processor or blender, purée the soup in batches. Season with salt and pepper.
7. Serve immediately.

Avocado Broccoli Soup

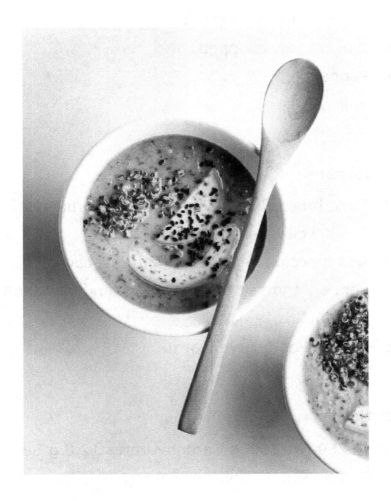

Preparation Time: 20 minutes

Cooking Time: 5 minutes

Servings: 4

Ingredients:

- 2 cups broccoli florets, chopped
- 5 cups vegetable broth
- 2 avocados, chopped
- Pepper
- Salt

Directions:

1. Cook broccoli in boiling water for 5 minutes. Drain well.
2. Add broccoli, vegetable broth, avocados, pepper, and salt to the blender and blend until smooth.
3. Stir well and serve warm.

Nutrition:

Calories 269 Fat 21.5 g Carbohydrates 12.8 g Sugar 2.1 g Protein 9.2 g Cholesterol 0 mg

Zoodle Bolognese

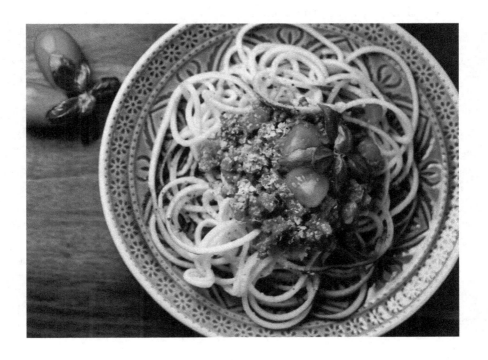

Preparation Time: 10minutes

Cooking Time: 35minutes

Serving: 4

Ingredients:

For the Bolognese sauce:

- 3 oz. olive oil
- 1 white onion, chopped

- 1 garlic clove, minced
- 3 oz. celery, chopped
- 3 cups crumbled tofu
- 2 tbsp tomato paste
- 1 ½ cups crushed tomatoes
- 1 tsp salt
- ¼ tsp black pepper
- 1 tbsp dried basil
- 1 tbsp Worcestershire sauce
- Water as needed

For the zoodles:

- 1 lb zucchinis
- 2 tbsp butter
- Salt and black pepper to taste

Directions:

1. Pour the olive oil into a saucepan and heat over medium heat. When no longer shimmering, add the onion, garlic, and celery. Sauté for 3 minutes or until the onions are soft and the carrots caramelized.
2. Pour in the tofu, tomato paste, tomatoes, salt, black pepper, basil, and Worcestershire sauce. Stir and cook for 15 minutes, or simmer for 30

minutes.

3. Mix in some water if the mixture is too thick and simmer further for 20 minutes.
4. While the sauce cooks, make the zoodles. Run the zucchini through a spiralizer to form noodles.
5. Melt the butter in a skillet over medium heat and toss the zoodles quickly in the butter, about 1 minute only.
6. Season with salt and black pepper.

Nutrition:

Calories: ,239 Total Fat:14.7g, Saturated Fat:8.1g, Total Carbs: 14g, Dietary Fiber:1g, Sugar:7 g, Protein: 13g, Sodium: 530mg

Delicious Sambal Seitan Noodles

Preparation Time: 60 minutes

Serving: 4

Ingredients:

For the shirataki noodles:

- 2 (8 oz) packs Miracle noodles, garlic and herb
- Salt to season

For the sambal seitan:

- 1 tbsp olive oil
- 1 lb seitan
- 4 garlic cloves, minced
- 1-inch ginger, peeled and grated
- 1 tsp liquid erythritol
- 1 tbsp sugar-free tomato paste
- 2 fresh basil leaves + extra for garnishing
- 2 tbsp sambal oelek
- 2 tbsp plain vinegar
- 1 cup water
- 2 tbsp coconut aminos
- Salt to taste

- 1 tbsp unsalted butter

Directions:

For the shirataki noodles:

1. Bring 2 cups of water to a boil in a medium pot over medium heat.
2. Strain the Miracle noodles through a colander and rinse very well under hot running water.
3. Allow proper draining and pour the noodles into the boiling water. Cook for 3 minutes and strain again.
4. Place a dry skillet over medium heat and stir-fry the shirataki noodles until visibly dry, 1 to 2 minutes. Season with salt, plate and set aside.

For the seitan sambal:

5. Heat the olive oil in a large pot and cook in the seitan until brown, 5 minutes.
6. Stir in the garlic, ginger, liquid erythritol and cook for 1 minute.
7. Add the tomato paste, cook for 2 minutes and mix in the basil, sambal oelek, vinegar, water, coconut aminos, and salt.

8. Cover the pot and continue cooking over low heat for 30 minutes.
9. Uncover, add the shirataki noodles, butter and mix well into the sauce.
10. Dish the food, garnish with some basil leaves and serve warm.

Nutrition:

Calories:538, Total Fat:41.1g, Saturated Fat:16.2g, Total Carbs:20g, Dietary Fiber:14g, Sugar:5g, Protein:29g, Sodium:640mg

Romaine And Grape Tomato Salad With Avocado And Baby Peas

Preparation time: 15 minutes

cooking time: 0 minutes

servings: 4

Ingredients

- 1 garlic clove, chopped
- 1 tablespoon chopped shallot
- 1/2 teaspoon dried basil
- 1/2 teaspoon salt
- 1/8 teaspoon freshly ground black pepper
- 1/4 teaspoon brown sugar (optional
- 3 tablespoons white wine vinegar
- 1/3 cup olive oil
- 1 medium head romaine lettuce, cut into 1/4-inch strips
- 12 ripe grape tomatoes, halved
- 1/2 cup frozen baby peas, thawed
- 8 kalamata olives, pitted
- 1 ripe Hass avocado

Directions

1. In a blender or food processor, combine the garlic, shallot, basil, salt, pepper, sugar, and vinegar until smooth. Add the oil and blend until emulsified. Set aside.

2. In a large bowl, combine the lettuce, tomatoes, peas, and olives. Pit and peel the avocado and cut into 1/2-inch dice. Add to the bowl, along with enough dressing to lightly coat. Toss gently to combine and serve.

Quick And Easy Ranch Dip

Preparation time: 10 minutes plus 4hrs chill time

Cooking time: 0 minutes

Servings: 12

Ingredients:

- 1 cup heavy (whipping) cream
- 1 tablespoon white distilled vinegar
- ¾ cup plain full-fat Greek yogurt
- 1 teaspoon freshly squeezed lemon juice
- 2 teaspoons dried parsley
- 1 teaspoon dried dill
- 1 teaspoon dried chives
- ½ teaspoon garlic powder
- ½ teaspoon onion powder
- ½ teaspoon salt
- ¼ teaspoon freshly ground black pepper

Directions:

1. In a quart-size canning jar, combine the heavy cream and vinegar. Set aside for 5 minutes.

2. Add the Greek yogurt and lemon juice and stir (or shake the jar) well.
3. Add the parsley, dill, chives, garlic powder, onion powder, salt, and pepper, and stir until thoroughly mixed.
4. Put the lid on the jar and place in the refrigerator for 4 hours or overnight for the flavors to combine.

Nutrition:

calories 79, fat 7g, protein 2g, carbs: 2g; fiber 0g, sugar 2g, sodium 109mg

Queso Blanco Dip

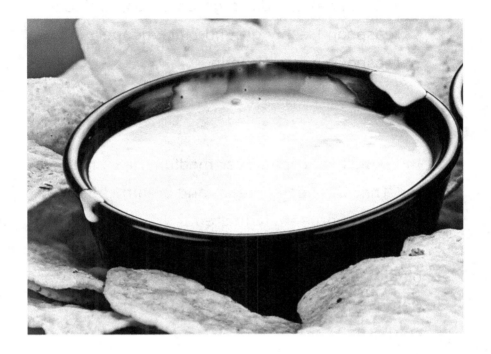

Preparation time: 5 minutes

Cooking time: 10 minutes

Servings: 8

Ingredients:

- ½ cup heavy (whipping) cream
- 3 ounces cream cheese
- 1 cup shredded Monterey Jack cheese

- 1 cup shredded queso blanco or other sharp white cheddar cheese
- 1 (4.5-ounce) can diced green chiles, drained
- ½ teaspoon freshly ground black pepper
- ½ teaspoon ground cumin

Directions:

1. In a small saucepan over medium heat, melt together the heavy cream and cream cheese, whisking until totally melted.
2. Stir in the Monterey Jack cheese and queso blanco and the green chiles.
3. Remove from the heat and add the pepper and cumin.
4. Stir well and serve.

Nutrition:

calories 202, fat 18g, protein 8g, carbs 2g, fiber 0g, sugar 1g, sodium 265mg

Tempeh-Pimiento Cheeze Ball

Preparation time: 5 minutes

cooking time: 30 minutes

servings: 8

Ingredients

- 8 ounces tempeh, cut into 1/2-inch pieces
- 1 (2-ouncejar chopped pimientos, drained
- 1/4 cup nutritional yeast
- 1/4 cup vegan mayonnaise, homemade or store-bought
- 2 tablespoons soy sauce
- ¾ cup chopped pecans

Directions

1. In a medium saucepan of simmering water, cook the tempeh for 30 minutes. Set aside to cool. In a food processor, combine the cooled tempeh, pimientos, nutritional yeast, mayo, and soy sauce. Process until smooth.

2. Transfer the tempeh mixture to a bowl and refrigerate until firm and chilled, at least 2 hours or overnight.

3. In a dry skillet, toast the pecans over medium heat until lightly toasted, about 5 minutes. Set aside to cool.

4. Shape the tempeh mixture into a ball, and roll it in the pecans, pressing the nuts slightly into the tempeh mixture so they stick. Refrigerate for at least 1 hour before serving. If not using right away, cover and keep refrigerated until needed. Properly stored, it will keep for 2 to 3 days.

Coconut Rice

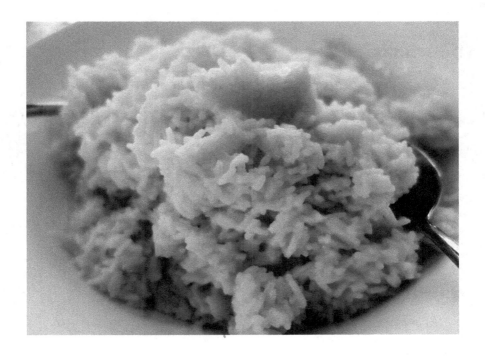

Preparation Time: 5 minutes

Cooking Time: 20 minutes

Servings: 4

Ingredients:

- 1 1/2 cups white rice
- 1 teaspoon coconut sugar
- 1/8 teaspoon salt

- 14 ounces coconut milk, unsweetened
- 1 1/4 cups water

Directions:

1. Take a saucepan, place it over medium heat, add all the ingredients in it, stir well and bring the mixture to a boil.
2. Switch heat to medium-low level, simmer the rice for 20 minutes until tender, and then serve straight away.

Nutrition:

Calories:453 Cal, Fat: 21 g, Carbs: 61.4 g, Protein: 6.8 g, Fiber: 2 g

Rice Pizza

Preparation Time: 10 minutes

Cooking Time: 35 minutes

Servings: 6

Ingredients:

For the crust:

- 1 1/2 cup short-grain rice, cooked
- 1/2 teaspoon garlic powder
- 1 teaspoon coconut sugar
- 1 tablespoon red chili flakes

For the sauce:

- 1/4 teaspoon onion powder
- 1 tablespoon nutritional yeast
- 1/4 teaspoon garlic powder
- 1/4 teaspoon ginger powder
- 1 tablespoon red chili flakes
- 1 teaspoon soy sauce
- 1/2 cup tomato purée

For the toppings:

- 2 1/2 cups oyster mushrooms
- 1 chili pepper, deseeded, sliced

- 2 scallions, sliced
- 1 teaspoon coconut sugar
- 1 teaspoon soy sauce
- Baby corn as needed

Directions:

1. Prepare the crust and for this, place all of its ingredients in a bowl and stir until well combined.
2. Then take a pizza pan, line it with parchment sheet, place rice mixture in it, spread it evenly, and then bake for 20 minutes at 350 degrees f.
3. Then spread tomato sauce over the crust, top evenly with remaining ingredients for the topping and continue baking for 15 minutes.
4. When done, slice the pizza into wedges and serve.

Nutrition:

Calories: 1 Cal, Fat: 5 g, Carbs: 30 g, Protein: 3 g, Fiber: 1 g

Quinoa and Black Bean Burgers

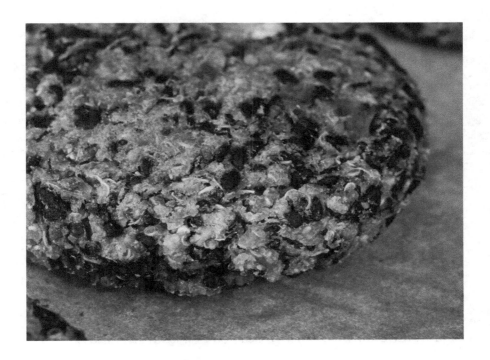

Preparation Time: 10 minutes

Cooking Time: 6 minutes

Servings: 5

Ingredients:

- 1/4 cup quinoa, cooked
- 15 ounces cooked black beans
- 2 tablespoons minced white onion

- 1/4 cup minced bell pepper
- ½ teaspoon minced garlic
- 1/2 teaspoon salt
- 1 1/2 teaspoons ground cumin
- 1/2 cup breadcrumbs
- 1 teaspoon hot pepper sauce
- 3 tablespoons olive oil
- 1 flax egg

Directions:

1. Place all the ingredients in a bowl, except for oil, stir until well combined, and then shape the mixture into five patties.
2. Heat oil in a frying pan over medium heat, add patties and cook for 3 minutes per side until browned.
3. Serve straight away.

Nutrition:

Calories: 245 Cal, Fat: 10.6 g, Carbs: 29 g, Protein: 9.3 g, Fiber: 7.2 g

Cinnamon Bun Balls

Preparation Time: 15 minutes

Cooking Time: 0 minute

Servings: 10

Ingredients:

- 5 medjool dates, pitted
- 1/2 cup whole walnuts
- 1 tablespoon chopped walnuts
- 3 tablespoons ground cinnamon
- 1 teaspoon ground cardamom

Directions:

1. Place all the ingredients in a food processor, except for 1 tablespoon walnuts, and then process until smooth.
2. Shape the mixture into ten balls, then roll them into chopped walnuts and serve.

Nutrition:

Calories:62 Cal, Fat: 4.5 g, Carbs: 5.8 g, Protein: 1.2 g, Fiber: 2 g

Strawberry Shortcake Chaffle Bowls

Preparation Time: 10 minutes

Cooking Time: 28 minutes

Servings: 4

Ingredients:

- 1 egg, beaten
- ½ cup finely grated mozzarella cheese
- 1 tbsp almond flour
- ¼ tsp baking powder
- 2 drops cake batter extract
- 1 cup cream cheese, softened
- 1 cup fresh strawberries, sliced
- 1 tbsp sugar-free maple syrup

Directions:

1. Preheat the cast iron pan.
2. Meanwhile, in a medium bowl, whisk all the ingredients except the cream cheese and strawberries.
3. Open the iron, pour in half of the mixture, cover, and cook until crispy, 6 to 7 minutes.

4. Remove the chaffle bowl onto a plate and set aside.
5. Make a second chaffle bowl with the remaining batter.
6. To serve, divide the cream cheese into the chaffle bowls and top with the strawberries.
7. Drizzle the filling with the maple syrup and serve.

Nutrition:

Calories 235, Fats 20.62g, Carbs 5.9g, Net Carbs 5g, Protein 7.51g

Mint Chocolate Chip Sorbet

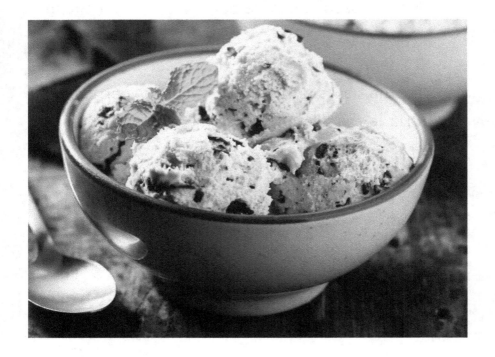

Preparation time: 5 minutes

cooking time: 0 minutes

servings: 1

Ingredients

- 1 frozen banana
- 1 tablespoon almond butter, or peanut butter, or other nut or seed butter

- 2 tablespoons fresh mint, minced
- ¼ cup or less non-dairy milk (only if needed
- 2 to 3 tablespoons non-dairy chocolate chips, or cocoa nibs
- 2 to 3 tablespoons goji berries (optional)

Directions

1. Put the banana, almond butter, and mint in a food processor or blender and purée until smooth.
2. Add the non-dairy milk if needed to keep blending (but only if needed, as this will make the texture less solid). Pulse the chocolate chips and goji berries (if using) into the mix so they're roughly chopped up.

Nutrition

Calories: 212; Total fat: 10g; Carbs: 31g; Fiber: 4g; Protein: 3g

Tangerine Stew

Preparation time: 10 minutes

Cooking time: 10 minutes

Servings: 4

Ingredients:

- 1 cup coconut water
- 2 cups tangerines, peeled and cut into segments
- 1 tablespoon lime juice
- 1 tablespoon stevia
- ½ teaspoon vanilla extract

Directions:

1. In a pan, combine the coconut water with the tangerines and the other ingredients, toss, bring to a simmer and cook over medium heat for 10 minutes.
2. Divide into bowls and serve cold.

Nutrition:

calories 289, fat 26.1, fiber 3.9, carbs 10.3, protein 5.7

Pineapple and Melon Stew

Preparation time: 10 minutes

Cooking time: 15 minutes

Servings: 4

Ingredients:

- 2 tablespoons stevia
- 1 cup pineapple, peeled and cubed
- 1 cup melon, peeled and cubed
- 2 cups water
- 1 teaspoon vanilla extract

Directions:

1. In a pan, combine the pineapple with the melon and the other ingredients, toss gently, cook over medium-low heat for 15 minutes, divide into bowls and serve cold.

Nutrition:

calories 40, fat 4.3, fiber 2.3, carbs 3.4, protein 0.8

Avocado and Rhubarb Salad

Preparation time: 10 minutes

Cooking time: 0 minutes

Servings: 4

Ingredients:

- 1 tablespoon stevia
- 1 cup rhubarb, sliced and boiled
- 2 avocados, peeled, pitted and sliced
- 1 teaspoon vanilla extract
- Juice of 1 lime

Directions:

1. In a bowl, combine the rhubarb with the avocado and the other ingredients, toss and serve.

Nutrition:

calories 140, fat 2, fiber 2, carbs 4, protein 4

Vanilla Raspberries Mix

Preparation time: 10 minutes

Cooking time: 10 minutes

Servings: 4

Ingredients:

- 1 cup water
- 1 cup raspberries
- 3 tablespoons stevia
- 1 teaspoon nutmeg, ground
- ½ teaspoon vanilla extract

Directions:

1. In a pan, combine the raspberries with the water and the other ingredients, toss, cook over medium heat for 10 minutes, divide into bowls and serve.

Nutrition:

calories 20, fat 0.4, fiber 2.1, carbs 4, protein 0.4

Sweet Zucchini Buns

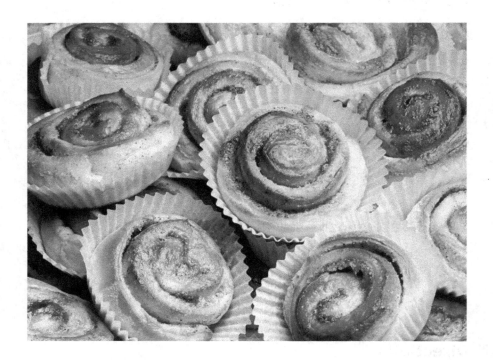

Preparation time: 10 minutes

Cooking time: 30 minutes

Servings: 8

Ingredients:

- 1 cup almond flour
- 1/3 cup coconut flesh, unsweetened and shredded

- 1 cup zucchinis, grated
- 2 tablespoons stevia
- 1 teaspoon baking soda
- ½ teaspoon cinnamon powder
- 3 tablespoons flaxseed mixed with 4 tablespoons water
- 1 cup coconut cream

Directions:

1. In a bowl, mix the almond flour with the coconut flesh, the zucchinis and the other ingredients, stir well until you obtain a dough, shape 8 buns and arrange them on a baking sheet lined with parchment paper.
2. Introduce in the oven at 350 degrees and bake for 30 minutes.
3. Serve these sweet buns warm.

Nutrition:

calories 169, fat 15.3, fiber 3.9, carbs 6.4, protein 3.2

Lime Berries Stew

Preparation time: 10 minutes

Cooking time: 20 minutes

Servings: 6

Ingredients:

- Zest of 1 lime, grated
- Juice of 1 lime
- 1 pint strawberries, halved
- 2 cups water
- 2 tablespoons stevia

Directions:

1. In a pan, combine the strawberries with the lime juice, the water and stevia, toss, bring to a simmer and cook over medium heat for 20 minutes.
2. Divide the stew into bowls and serve cold.

Nutrition:

calories 172, fat 7, fiber 3.4, carbs 8, protein 2.3

Apricots Cake

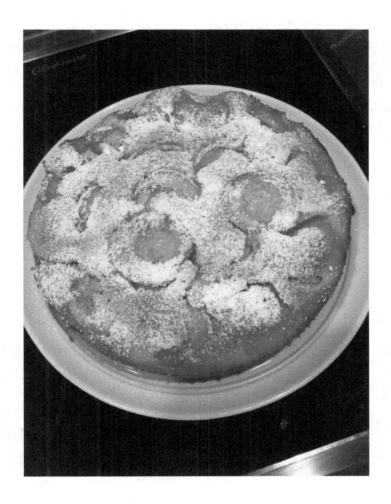

Preparation time: 10 minutes

Cooking time: 30 minutes

Servings: 8

Ingredients:

- ¾ cup stevia
- 2 cups coconut flour
- ¼ cup coconut oil, melted
- ½ cup almond milk
- 1 teaspoon baking powder
- 2 tablespoons flaxseed mixed with 3 tablespoons water
- ½ teaspoon vanilla extract
- Juice of 1 lime
- 2 cups apricots, chopped

Directions:

1. In a bowl, mix the flour with the coconut oil, the stevia and the other ingredients, whisk and pour into a cake pan lined with parchment paper.
2. Introduce in the oven at 375 degrees F, bake for 30 minutes, cool down, slice and serve.

Nutrition:

calories 221, fat 8.3, fiber 3.4, carbs 14.5, protein 5

Nutmeg Pudding

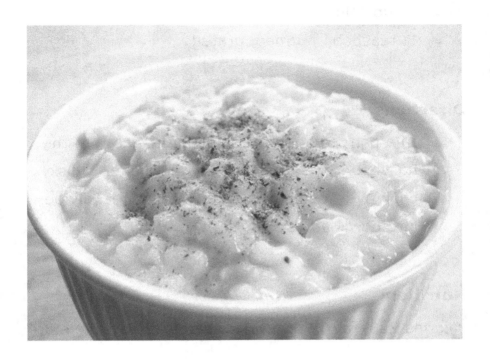

Preparation time: 10 minutes

Cooking time: 20 minutes

Servings: 6

Ingredients:

- 2 tablespoons stevia
- 1 teaspoon nutmeg, ground
- 1 cup cauliflower rice

- 2 tablespoons flaxseed mixed with 3 tablespoons water
- 2 cups almond milk
- ¼ teaspoon nutmeg, grated

Directions:

1. In a pan, combine the cauliflower rice with the flaxseed mix and the other ingredients, whisk, cook over medium heat for 20 minutes, divide into bowls and serve cold.

Nutrition:

calories 220, fat 6.6, fiber 3.4, carbs 12.4, protein 3.4

Avocado and Almond Sweet Cream

Preparation time: 20 minutes

Cooking time: 0 minutes

Servings: 6

Ingredients:

- 2 avocados, peeled, pitted and mashed
- 1 cup coconut cream
- 2 tablespoons stevia
- 1 teaspoon almond extract
- ¾ cup stevia
- ¾ cup almonds, ground

Directions:

1. In a blender, combine the avocados with the cream and the other ingredients, pulse well, divide into cups and keep in the fridge for at least 20 minutes before serving.

Nutrition:

calories 106, fat 3.4, fiber 0, carbs 2.4, protein 4

Chia Bowls

Preparation time: 5 minutes

Cooking time: 0 minutes

Servings: 2

Ingredients:

- 2 cups coconut milk, warm
- ½ cup coconut cream
- 1 cup cauliflower rice, steamed
- 2 tablespoons stevia
- 2 tablespoons chia seeds
- 1 teaspoon cinnamon powder

Directions:

1. In a bowl, combine the cream with the milk, the cauliflower rice and the other ingredients, whisk, well, leave aside for 5 minutes, divide into small bowls and serve cold.

Nutrition:

calories 182, fat 3.4, fiber 3.4, carbs 8.4, protein 3

Cocoa Cream

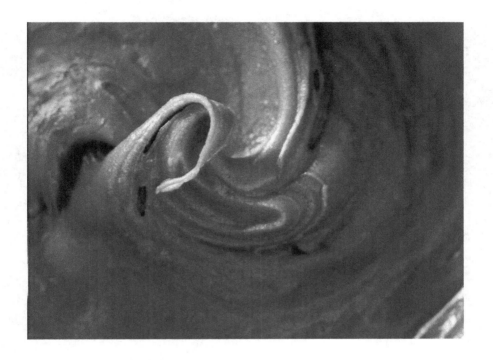

Preparation time: 2 hours

Cooking time: 0 minutes

Servings: 4

Ingredients:

- ½ cup cocoa powder
- ¾ cup coconut cream
- ¼ cup stevia

- 1 teaspoon cinnamon powder
- 1 teaspoon vanilla extract

Directions:

1. In a blender, mix the cream with the cocoa powder, stevia and the other ingredients, pulse well, divide into cups and keep in the fridge for 2 hours before serving.

Nutrition:

calories 162, fat 3.4, fiber 2.4, carbs 5, protein 1

Raspberry Protein Shake (vegan)

Preparation Time: 5 minutes

Cooking Time: 0 minute

Servings: 2

Ingredients:

- 1 cup full-fat coconut milk (or alternatively, use almond milk)
- Optional: ¼ cup coconut cream
- 1 scoop organic soy protein (chocolate or vanilla flavor)
- ½ cup raspberries (fresh or frozen)
- 1 tbsp. low-carb maple syrup
- Optional: 2-4 ice cubes

Directions:

1. Add all the ingredients to a blender, including the optional coconut cream and ice cubes if desired, and blend for 1 minute.
2. Transfer the shake to a large cup or shaker, and enjoy!

3. Alternatively, store the smoothie in an airtight container or a mason jar, keep it in the fridge, and consume within 2 days. Store for a maximum of 30 days in the freezer and thaw at room temperature.

Nutrition:

Calories: 311kcal, Net carbs: 4.6g, Fat: 25.7g, Protein: 14.65g, Fiber: 3.5g, Sugar: 3.35g

NOTE

CPSIA information can be obtained
at www.ICGtesting.com
Printed in the USA
BVHW091921230621
610293BV00007B/851